Dr. Walter Reed – A Short Biography

By Erin DeLong

Dr. Walter Reed – A Short Biography

Copyright © 2015 Erin DeLong

All Rights Reserved. No part of this book may be reproduced in any form without written permission from the author. Reviewers may quote brief passages in reviews.

Table of Contents

Preface

Welcome to the book *Dr. Walter Reed – A Short Biography*. This book is part of the *30 Minute Book Series* and, as the name of the series implies, if you are an average reader this book will take around 30 minutes to read or a little longer to listen to in audio format. Since this book is not meant to be an all-encompassing biography of Dr. Walter Reed, you may want to know more about this great doctor and his accomplishments. To help you with this, there are several good references at the end of this book. Thank you for purchasing this book and I hope you enjoy your time reading about this amazing doctor and scientist.

Erin DeLong

October 2015

Introduction

Walter Reed. Chances are, you are familiar with his name only because you have heard of the major army medical center named after him. Maybe you have heard of his name in general references related to yellow fever. Either way, there is so much more to this humble, hard-working man than most know. He wore many hats, and husband, father, military officer, scientist, and doctor are just a few. Some of his scientific achievements are benefiting humanity today. To truly understand the depth of accomplishment by Dr. Walter Reed, you must first value the scourge he helped unravel: yellow fever.

Yellow fever had been a mystery since the fifteenth century, when its first cases were documented; some even believe that yellow fever was the cause of death for many of Christopher Columbus's men. It affected the people of the United States annually. Initially, more people living in the southern states were impacted, but as railroad and steamboat transportation flourished, this disease began to pop up in more northern areas. People knew what time of the year yellow fever was likely to emerge, during what temperature and weather conditions, and in what part of the United States, but no one could discover the missing links of how or why.

Imagine the fear as family members began to fall ill with yellow fever. Mom would get it, but not Dad. Two out of three children might get it. Yellow fever would sweep into the poorer sections of town but also strike the more affluent areas. Many of the tenements, as well as hospitals, would see yellow fever epidemics. It didn't seem to matter if people burned everything in their house or bought the highest quality items;

it did not make them immune to the ravages of this disease. It might kill a city by the thousands one year and be nearly absent in that city the next year. In just two or three months, yellow fever could kill twenty percent of a city's population. People were terrified.

With the limited medical knowledge of that period of time and the patterns of yellow fever striking, scientists were perplexed as they could not figure out the illness. Meanwhile, thousands of lives were lost to the mysterious illness. Panic would strike the city. Businesses would close and people would move out of the city in fear. Some cities went bankrupt during such terror. Bridges were literally burned so travelers could not enter into their city and possibly bring this strange illness. Some travelers would receive a shotgun warning to not enter their city. People were stricken with terror and would go to great lengths to protect their families and livelihoods. However, the long reign of panic from this illness was about to end.

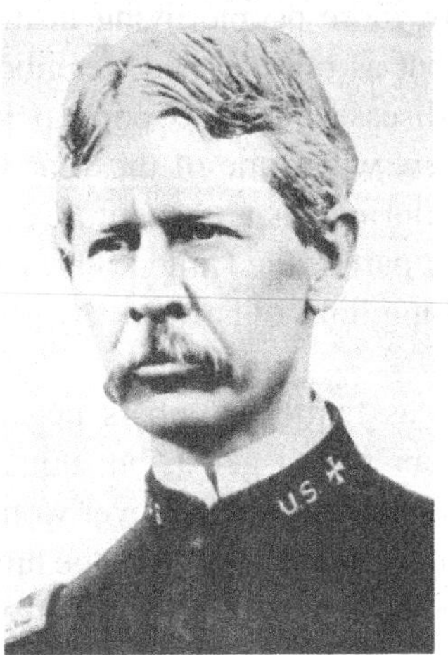

Figure – Walter Reed

CHAPTER 1

The Early Years

Our story begins in a small, modest parsonage in Virginia. In just a two bedroom home, built in the first half of the nineteenth century, the youngest of five children, Walter Reed, was born on September 13, 1851, in Gloucester County. Lemuel Sutton Reed and Pharaba White, as well as Laura, James, Thomas, and Christopher Reed welcomed him into the family. His father was a Methodist minister who spent his life devoted to the church and his family. Rather than wealth and worldly pleasures, the Reeds valued service, integrity, and morality. This moral code and lifestyle would prove beneficial, as the Reed children matured into adults with successful career paths.

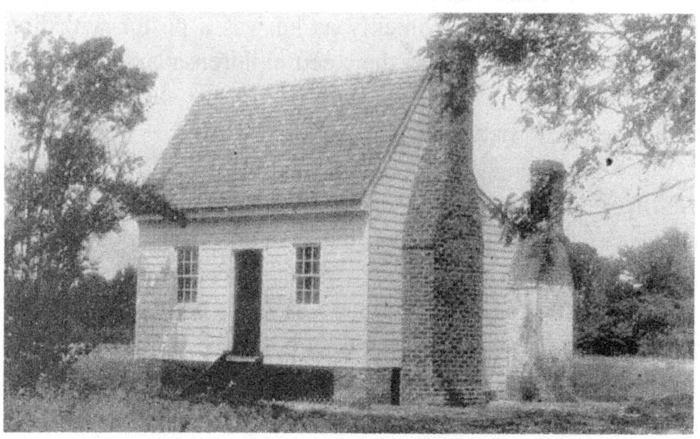

Figure – Walter Reed's Birth Home

Throughout Walter's childhood, he spent much time moving due to his father's career. As was normal for Methodist ministers, the family transferred every few years to a new parsonage. When Walter was only fourteen months old, he experienced his first move when his family was relocated to another part of the state. Throughout his childhood, the family resided in several communities in North Carolina and Virginia. When Walter was nine years old, the Civil War began and two of his brothers served in the Confederacy. This was a precarious time in that part of the nation, and it would prove dangerous and risky to the family. However, by the end of the war, everyone's life was spared and the only family casualty was his brother James's hand.

Shortly after the Civil War, Walter's family settled in Charlottesville, Virginia. Around this time, another hardship impacted his family. Pharaba White, Walter's mother, became gravely ill and died. This was devastating to a fourteen year old Walter Reed. Characteristic of this time period, Lemuel Reed remarried rather quickly as he was a pastor with five children. Life changed as the Reed children adapted to their new stepmother, Mary Catherine Byrd. In a short period of time, their new sister, Anna, was born, in 1867.

Living in Charlottesville during this time had been at the request of Lemuel Reed, so that his sons could begin more formal studies. Growing up, Walter Reed's education was considered normal for the time period, as some of it was in public school and some of it was at home. He studied English, Latin, Greek, history, humanities, and other traditional areas of learning. Some might say he was a bit of a prodigy.

CHAPTER 2

Becoming a Doctor

At 16, Walter began school at the nearby University of Virginia, where his brothers, James and Christopher, also attended. After the first year of Walter's studies, it became evident that the financial burden of three sons in a university was too expensive for Walter's father. Walter took it upon himself to work towards a medical degree since it would be quicker to complete than a Master's degree. Walter also challenged the school to award him his degree earlier if he could pass all the necessary exams to become a doctor. With hard work and conviction, Walter passed all of his exams before his 18th birthday. In a class of 50, he was ranked third. He received his Doctor of Medicine in 1869 and remains the youngest person to graduate from the University of Virginia Medical School to this day.

After his graduation, Walter still desired further study in the medical profession so he moved to New York to study at the Bellevue Hospital Medical College. There he would earn a second degree. For several years, Walter Reed interned in New York in several different hospitals. He was an Assistant Physician at New York Infants' Hospital, an Assistant Physician at Kings County Hospital, and a Resident Surgeon at Brooklyn City Hospital. During this time, Walter Reed also served as a District Physician for the New York Department of Public Charities. His young age, compassionate heart, and sharp mind provided him many different opportunities. These valuable opportunities would help him gain much needed experience as he began to define the direction he wanted his medical career to go.

At the age of 22, Walter was appointed a job with the Brooklyn Board of Health as a Sanitation Inspector. There were only five inspectors at the time. This particular job gave Walter much insight into neighborhoods that were full of densely populated tenements. Some say this is where his love for public health was sparked. About his time in New York, Walter Reed wrote, "My stay in these cities has done me an incomparable goode. By it I have obtained an extensive hospital and sanitary experience which is worth to me more than I can now estimate. It has also given me a truer insight into human nature than I would have acquired in an equal number of years elsewhere, while it has added to my respect for truth and morality. So that I count myself more than fortunate so far."

During a series of visits home to see his family, who were then living in Murfreesboro, Virginia, Walter Reed met a very special person, Emilie Lawrence. It wasn't long until they began officially courting, mainly through letters as Walter was still living and working in New York. When it became apparent to him that he would one day marry Emilie, Walter felt that he must find consistent work to sustain his future wife and a family. Walter was ready for a life outside of the large metropolis. His solution to achieving his desires was to join the Army Medical Corps.

Joining the medical corps was not easy, as he had to pass a very challenging examination. The exam consisted of information about a wide range of medical topics but also Latin, Greek, mathematics, and history. Walter had to spend a lot of time preparing and studying for this arduous 30 hour exam that was given over six successive days. Not only did he have to pass the exam, but there were five hundred applicants, at the time, and less than thirty vacancies. He wrote to his dear Emilie during this time, describing the great strain he felt about this rigorous exam. However, his intelligence and resolve prevailed again. He passed the examinations and on June 26, 1875, he was appointed Assistant Surgeon in the United States Army.

CHAPTER 3

Life as an Officer

His first duty station was at Willet's Point in New York, which was one of the most sought after posts. Walter Reed wrote to Emilie describing his days as rather easy. He would attend to the soldiers at "sick call" in the morning and then make rounds at the hospital. There weren't many patients, however, and Walter was afforded much free time.

Meanwhile, back in Murfreesboro, Emilie Lawrence was busy planning their wedding. Walter's "plush" life as a new lieutenant didn't last long as he received word that he would soon be moving to his next duty station in Fort Lowell, Arizona. Walter quickly notified Emilie of his new duty station and their wedding date was moved up. On April 26, Walter and Emilie were married in Murfreesboro in the same church in which they had first met. Lemuel Reed officiated the ceremony. No one, including themselves, could have imagined the life and travels they were getting ready to embark on!

In 1876, their first duty station sent them to Arizona, which may have felt like half a world away, especially for a young married couple who had lived most of their lives up north. This was considered a frontier that was not as established as the northern states in which they had resided. At this time, the West was still rough and practically uncivilized. It had been less than 10 years since the completion of the transcontinental railroad. Life was not easy on the frontier.

Walter Reed initially moved to Arizona without his new bride. In a few months, Emilie traveled from Virginia to San Francisco, where the couple reunited to travel back to their new home in Arizona. It was during the separation from Emilie that Walter Reed grew a thick mustache, which he then kept the rest of his life. Perhaps this mustache represented Walter's step into his new adult life as an officer and husband.

It took the couple more than three weeks to travel 500 miles over rough terrain in a wagon to get to Fort Lowell, Arizona. One can only imagine the bumpiness and roughness of the road day after day, only to find relief camping out in the open Wild West at night. It was quite a trek and most likely not the dream or fantasy of any newly married couple. However, the Reeds approached this journey together with determination and optimism. Once the newlyweds arrived in Arizona, they discovered that temperatures were often in excess of 100 degrees Fahrenheit and that the landscape was dusty and barren. Everything in their life was drastically changed as they were getting their first doses of "frontier life."

This new duty station and its responsibilities were completely different from Walter's time at Willet's Point in New York. While in New York, he had a relatively small patient load. Now, at times, he was the only physician in over 200 miles. He was now responsible for providing care to soldiers, dependents, civilians, and Indians. If someone needed medical help in the area, they went to Dr. Reed. Due to the frontier not being civilized, medical supplies and equipment were not readily available. He often had few supplies and primitive instruments as he attempted to give his varied patients the very best care possible.

Over the next decade, Walter Reed was sent to many different garrison posts around Arizona, Nebraska, Minnesota, and Alabama. Many of the posts were located in remote areas and Walter Reed was practicing frontier medicine, which was a very practical form of medicine. While moving frequently and living in these frontier locations, Walter and Emilie were blessed with children, most likely delivered in their home with his assistance. Emilie and Walter had a son named Walter Lawrence Reed, who was born on December 4, 1877, while they were stationed at Fort Apache in Arizona. A few years later, their daughter, Emilie Reed, who went by Blossom, was born in Omaha, Nebraska, in 1883.

During the course of their stay at Camp Apache, Arizona, the Reeds also informally adopted a young Indian girl by the name of Susie, who was probably four or five years old at the time. Susie's family abandoned her due to severe burns and she was brought to Dr. Reed for care. Dr. Reed and Emilie operated on their integrity, and with family values being cornerstone, it seemed instinctive to bring this young girl into their home and raise her. As Walter and Emilie tended to her needs and nursed her back to health, Susie became a part of their family. She lived and traveled with them for the next 15 years. After Susie became a young adult, she was able to return to her Indian roots, and contact with the Reed family broke off.

Walter Reed's continual hard work, dedication, and flexibility earned him what he needed for his next promotion. On June 26, 1880, he was promoted to captain. After his promotion he was transferred to Fort McHenry in Baltimore, Maryland. While Reed's work allowed for a great deal of professional growth, he realized his line of work was not allowing him to do any research or learn of medical advancements. While at Fort McHenry, Reed was able to attend many fascinating lectures at John Hopkins University on the emerging field of bacteriology. This time of educational refreshment did not last long as the Reed family were moved to another duty station.

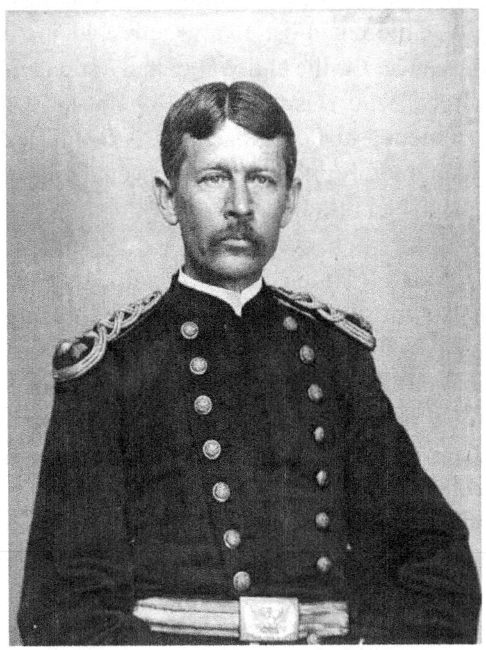

Figure – Walter Reed in Uniform

Ten more years of frontier travel would occur for Walter Reed and his family. Year by year, the fields of bacteriology and pathology continued to grow and develop. Scientific discoveries were being made and the science and practice of medicine was moving forward, and all the while Walter Reed was still traveling and practicing antiquated medicine with little provision.

While back in Baltimore, in 1890, Walter Reed received permission to enroll and study at John Hopkins University, where he would be able to learn more about the emerging field of bacteriology. At that time, bacteriology was defined as the study of bacteria and its relation to medicine and other areas of agriculture and industry. He studied under a distinguished teacher, William H. Welch, who was a former student of Louis Pasteur and Director of the Pathology laboratory. At the time of Walter's initial studies in the medical field, bacteriology and pathology were not part of the curriculum. Therefore, many of the techniques and methods that Walter learned during this time would prove crucial to his studies and experiments later on in his medical career. Also during his time at John Hopkins, Walter Reed first met Dr. James Carroll, a United States Army physician also studying there, who would become a research partner and close friend.

CHAPTER 4

Life in Washington, DC

Walter Reed was promoted to Major on December 4, 1893, and was moved to Washington, DC. The Surgeon General of the United States, George Sternberg, appointed Reed as the curator of the Army Medical Museum and a Professor of Clinical and Sanitary Microscopy and Director of Pathological Laboratory at the new Army Medical College. His appointments to these positions would offer him invaluable opportunities for learning and research that would contribute to other scientific findings later in life.

After a few years in Washington, DC, Walter was given the opportunity to unravel his first medical mystery. Malaria was a widespread problem at the Washington Barracks and at Fort Myer in Virginia. At this time, it was widely believed that malaria was caused by bad drinking water. However, in these outbreaks, it seemed to largely affect the enlisted men and not the officers, even though both groups of men drank the same water and had a similar diet. Dr. Walter Reed decided to explore a more sociological, rather than scientific, route on his investigation, and began to analyze and question the behaviors and habits of these two groups of men. After some inquiring, he found out that the enlisted men were sneaking out at night to explore the city. They would creep back to base by taking a trail through the marshlands of the Potomac River. He was not able to identify the route in which malaria was transmitted, but he was able to identify the behavior that was contributing to the breakout.

Five years into his time in Washington, DC, on April 25, 1898, the United States declared war on Spain following the sinking of the Battleship Maine in Havana Harbor. Secretary of State John Hay called it "the splendid little war," and little it was, lasting only four months. While the conflict was short, it represented years of struggle for Cuba. It only took a few major battles in Cuba and in the Pacific Ocean for the United States to come out triumphant. In December, the Treaty of Paris was signed by both countries, formally ending the war. However, the United States would still have a presence in Cuba, helping the new government establish itself and ensuring peace was maintained. At the conclusion of the war, approximately 50,000 American soldiers were still stationed in Cuba.

Disease would kill far more men during the Spanish American war than the combat itself. Approximately 968 men died to hostile fire while over 5,000 died to disease. Soldiers were dying in training camps in the United States as well as in Cuba. Sanitation and disease were an embarrassment to the United States military during this time. Walter Reed was appointed the chairman of the Typhoid Board by the Surgeon General in August 1898. Typhoid fever was being experienced in Army training camps in epidemic proportions. Typhoid fever is an acute illness that causes headache, cough, vomiting, and diarrhea, and about twenty percent of the cases will result in death. The Army camps were seeing hundreds of new cases of this every day; many of the cases ended up being fatal. Bad water was first believed to be the culprit; however, upon further investigation, it was found that the disease was being spread by flies and contact with fecal matter.

It took the Typhoid Board two years to fully identify the cause and support their findings. However, their results would prove invaluable in ending the epidemic the soldiers were experiencing. The combined research, discoveries, and recommendations would become a vast two volume report that would be used by epidemiologists for many years to come. The scientific approach and proposals included in this report would be a foundation for all future successful public health models.

After Dr. Reed's time on the Typhoid Board, he was appointed the head of another Army board to investigate the infectious diseases in Cuba, particularly yellow fever. This disease was ravaging the camps of soldiers in Cuba. For decades, scientists and medical professionals had been working to figure out the cause of yellow fever. Now Walter Reed had a chance to focus his efforts on the mystery of yellow fever. Several men had spent time before him studying this illness. Nearly 50 years before he was appointed on this board, a physician in Alabama, Josiah Nott, had proposed that yellow fever was caused by an insect, maybe even a mosquito, but had no substantial evidence to support his findings. Dr. Nott lost four of his children to yellow fever in one week. Twenty years before Walter Reed would begin his yellow fever work, another physician, Carlos Finlay, proposed that a specific mosquito, *Culex fasciatus*, transmitted yellow fever. He received widespread criticism and skepticism for his theory. Although he carried out several studies to try to prove his theories, he was never able to prove it with complete certainty.

As Walter Reed began his work on the illness of yellow fever, he would walk into a great debate that was underway. A younger Italian physician, Dr. Giuseppe Sanarelli, published a rather lengthy report stating that yellow fever was caused by *Bacillus icteroides*. Other physicians were in disagreement, such as an older, more experienced physician, the Army Surgeon General, Dr. George Miller Sternberg, who believed differently. That same year he published a report that claimed that *"Bacillis X"* was the causative agent of yellow fever. The scientific battle lines were drawn as the medical professionals tried to figure out the mysterious and often fatal disease. In the end, Dr. Walter Reed would prove that neither of these men were correct; rather, he would credit Carlos Finlay, who first proposed the theory that ended up being correct.

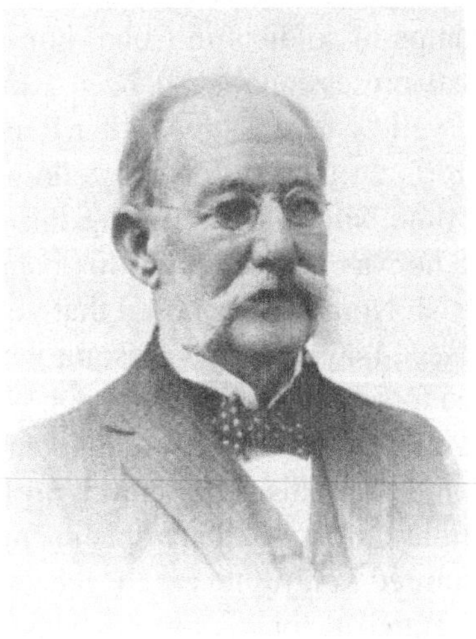

Figure – Carlos Finlay

CHAPTER 5

Yellow Fever Work Begins

In May of 1900, Surgeon General of the US Army, George Sternberg, appointed Walter Reed, along with James Carroll, Jesse Lazear, and Aristides Agramonte of Havana, as the US Army Yellow Fever Commission. Walter Reed was the head of the project, with Carroll being in charge of bacteriology, Lazear in charge of laboratory work, and Agramonte in charge of pathology. Carroll and Reed arrived in Cuba the next month, joining Agramonte and Lazear, and began their research together. Surprisingly, Walter Reed had never seen a yellow fever patient in his professional career. His first task, upon his arrival to Cuba, was to visit his personal friend, Major Jefferson R. Kean, Chief Surgeon of the Department of Western Cuba, who was ill in the hospital with yellow fever. This would be his first physical interaction with yellow fever.

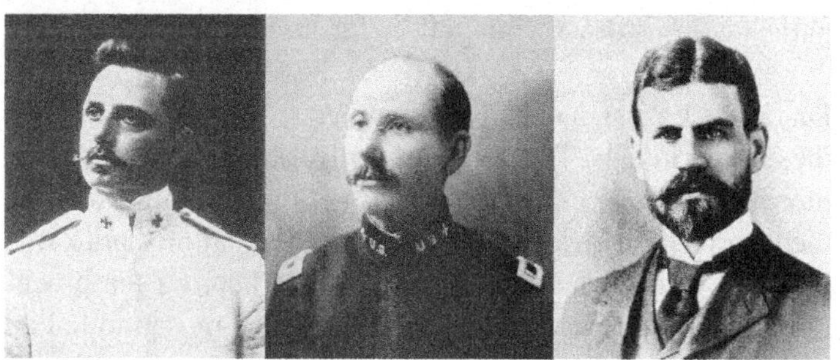

Figure – (From Left to Right – Aristides Agramonte, James Carroll, Jesse Lazear)

These brilliant men believed the best way to approach their research on yellow fever was not by searching for the causative agent, but rather by recognizing the route in which it was transmitted. This approach brought them back to the work of Carlos Finlay. The board members visited him at his home in Cuba to discuss his theories on yellow fever transmission by a female mosquito. After discussions with Finlay, the men decided to attempt Finlay's previous experimental trials but with much stricter laboratory controls in place. First they wanted to know how yellow fever was transmitted. Additionally they wished to disprove the theory that yellow fever could be spread by soiled items, such as clothing and linens. This belief had caused people to destroy everything in contact with this disease, wasting thousands of dollars.

After spending the summer there, in August Reed traveled back to Washington to tie up some loose ends with the Typhoid Board. The rest of the men continued with their work while he was gone. The first experiments to test Finlay's theories involved having mosquitoes feed on volunteers. The intention of this experiment was to have controlled proof of a patient coming down with yellow fever via a mosquito.

Dr. Jesse Lazear hatched mosquitoes from eggs to use for these experiments. To feed them, daily, Lazear would take the mosquitoes to the yellow fever ward of the hospital and allow them to feed on sick patients. Each individual mosquito was kept in a test tube. Meticulous data was kept on the procedures, such as which patient or patients each mosquito fed on and what stage of the illness the patient was in.

A cotton stopper was taken out of each test tube one by one, as the mosquito was allowed onto the patient's skin to feed. Once it was done, the mosquito would become airborne, alerting Lazear he was done. The cotton stopper was put back into place and Lazear would move onto the next mosquito. This "loading," as it was called, was what kept the Board's mosquitoes alive.

On the afternoon of August 27, Lazear noticed one mosquito had not "fed" and could quite possibly die. He expressed his concern to Carroll. Up until this point, nine volunteers had been used and not one "official" case of yellow fever had been confirmed through their experiments. The men were frustrated by this, and perhaps Carroll didn't feel threatened or concerned when considering whether he should volunteer or not. Perhaps Carroll was more concerned with the experiments moving forward. Either way, Carroll sacrificed himself for the cause, volunteered to have the mosquito feed on him, and then went on with his normal responsibilities, just as if nothing had happened. He did not quarantine himself, as was demanded of previous volunteers.

Two days later, it became clear that something had happened. Carroll became ill and the next day he was taken to the Columbia Barracks yellow fever wards. The following day it was confirmed he had come down with yellow fever. He was experiencing high fevers, jaundice, and delusions and was forced to stay in bed.

Yellow fever is a very unpleasant illness. It began with headache, chills, and fever, then it progressed to body aches, nausea and vomiting, back pain, fatigue, and weakness. The feverish stage might last hours, days, or weeks. Jaundice, a yellow hue on the body and eyes, may begin to appear; this symptom is where yellow fever derives its name. Then came the so-called "stage of calm," when the severity of the symptoms subsided and the fever declined. At this point, some would begin to recover. For some, however, the fever would come back with a vengeance, signaling the final stage of the illness. As yellow fever is a hemorrhagic fever, internal bleeding would be occurring at this point, causing the dreaded "black vomit." The patient would experience multiple organ failure, shock, and then death.

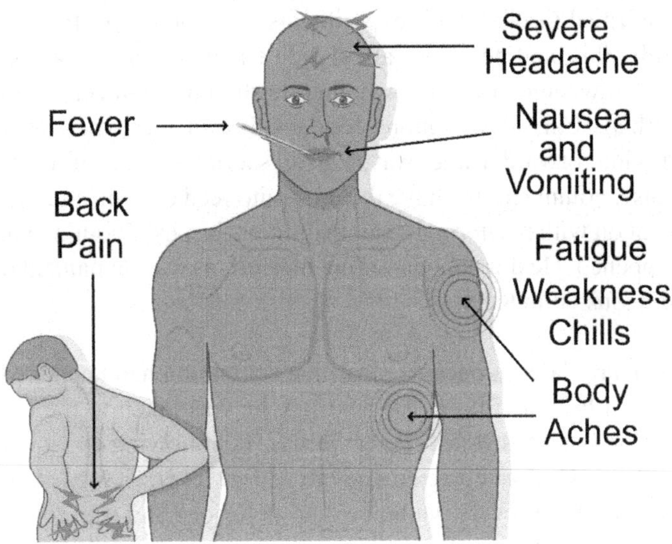

Figure – Signs and Symptoms of Yellow Fever

Although Carroll would be one of the lucky ones to recover, his recuperation would be a lengthy one. However, the experiments continued forward. Since Carroll had not been in quarantine, his contracting of yellow fever could not be proved irrefutably. Lazear began to look for another human volunteer. Lazear came across Private William Dean at the hospital one day and asked him if he would like to volunteer for some experiments involving mosquitoes. Lazear used the same mosquito that had infected Carroll and allowed it to feed on Private Dean. Agramonte wrote in an article for *Scientific Monthly*, entitled "The Inside of History of a Great Medical Discovery," published December 1915:

"…[To the soldier, Private Dean]…I asked him to come inside and bare his forearm. Upon a slip of paper I wrote his name while several mosquitoes took their fill: William H. Dean, American by birth, belonging to Troop B, Seventh Cavalry; he said that he had never been in the tropics before and had not left the military reservation for nearly two months. The conditions for a test case were quite ideal.

"I must say we were in great trepidation at the time; and well might we have been, for Dean's was the first indubitable case of yellow fever about to be produced experimentally by the bite of purposely infected mosquitoes. Five days afterwards, when he came down with yellow fever and the diagnosis of his case corroborated with Dr. Roger P. Ames, US Army, then on duty at the hospital, we sent a cablegram to Major Walter Reed, chairman of the board, who a month before had been called to Washington upon another duty, apprising him of the fact that the theory of the transmission of yellow fever by mosquitoes, which at first was doubted so much and the transcendental importance of which we could then barely appreciate, had indeed been confirmed."

This was indeed an amazing moment for the men. Dean's case of yellow fever was mild and he recovered quickly. Reed was eager to get back to Cuba, to see firsthand what was going on and also to check on his friend and colleague, Carroll, who was still recovering.

The next month, another board member, Jesse Lazear also became infected with yellow fever. Some believe he did this on purpose, in the name of scientific research. Some believe it was an accident, while he was completing his research. The real truth of how he contracted yellow fever, none of us will ever know. He became ill on September 18, and his illness progressed quickly to the final stage, where he exhibited convulsions, delirium, and black vomit. One September 25, Jesse Lazear died.

His death was a blow to the men, but his death was not in vain. He would be remembered for his work and ultimate sacrifice to science. Nonetheless, the scientific work and research had to go on. Reed arrived back in Cuba and threw himself into research. He scoured all the notebooks and information that Jesse Lazear had. During this time, Carroll was still recovering and Agramonte was on leave, so Reed was working on his own. In October, Reed was called back the United States to a meeting in Indianapolis. After some presentations and work in the United States, including visiting his family, Reed headed back to Cuba.

CHAPTER 6

Camp Lazear

Once back in Cuba, Walter Reed immediately went to work on plans for his final experiment. It would be done in Cuba, in a camp set away from any other people. Camp Lazear was established and named after their associate, Jesse Lazear, who had just died a few months prior. It opened on November 20, 1900. No yellow fever had been known to be in the area of Camp Lazear and it was clear of standing water and was open to the sun and wind. The camp was put under strict quarantine and two buildings were constructed for the trials.

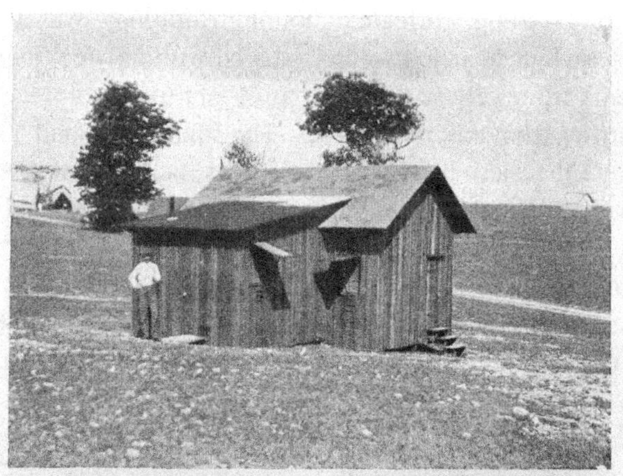

CAMP LAZEAR

Building where the experiments were made which proved that yellow fever is not transmitted by means of infected clothing (fomites)

Figure – Camp Lazear

Volunteers for the study were offered $100 in gold to partici-pate and an additional $100 in gold if they contracted yellow fever. They were promised to receive excellent medical care if they became ill. Additionally, the volunteers were required to give written consent. Although this is normal practice today, back then this was ground-breaking. It was not custom to re-ceive written consent on human volunteers and no regulations or guidelines existed on this kind of medical research. The US Army Yellow Fever Commission is considered to be the first group to use consent forms in its experiments. One of the first volunteers was Private John Kissinger, who denied any finan-cial compensation and stated he was participating for the sake of the greater good and for science. His courage to volunteer and come forward encouraged other soldiers to come forward as well, even though they were not explicitly recruited.

The first building, "Infected Clothing Building," was a small room in which selected soldiers stayed with only contaminat-ed items from yellow fever patients, and these soldiers were kept away from any mosquitoes. The small room had a stove that kept the room heated to 90-95 degrees Fahrenheit. Along the walls, contaminated linens and items were hung. Every night they slept in sheets that were dirty with vomit, blood, and other body fluids of patients ill with yellow fever. One of the volunteers, Dr. Robert Cooke, said, "We all felt like we were coming down with yellow fever every day." Though quite thoroughly exposed and probably very disgusted, none of these soldiers contracted the disease.

The second building, "Infected Mosquito Building," was sep-arated into two parts by a screen. On one side a participant was lying in a clean bed where several infected mosquitoes were released. On the other side of the screen the doctors viewed and recorded his mosquito bites. Additionally, other participants sat, breathing in the same air, but were not exposed to the infected mosquitoes.

Tests in the "Infected Mosquito Building" began on December 21, 1900. The first volunteer into the "Infected Mosquito Building" was John Moran. He wore only his nightshirt and lay down in the cot and was bitten by several mosquitoes. Four days after he had received his fifteen mosquito bites from the infected mosquito, on Christmas Day, he began experiencing symptoms of yellow fever. The participants on the mosquito-free side slept in the "Infected Mosquito Building" for eighteen more nights. None of them came down with yellow fever. During the course of the yellow fever experiments, several men contracted yellow fever, but all of them had a successful recovery.

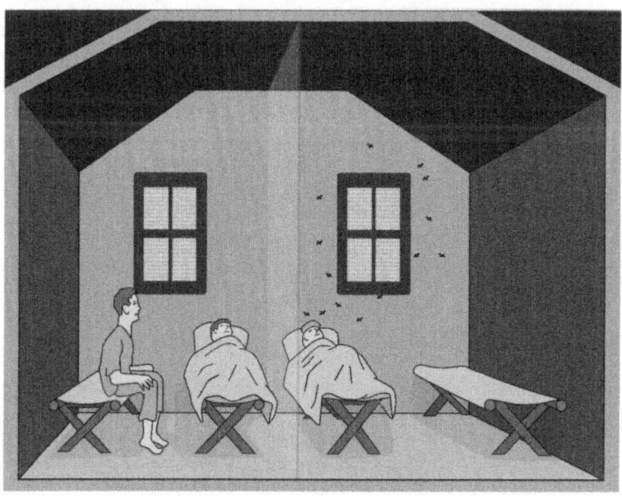

Figure – Infected Mosquito Building

The main finding of the studies in Cuba was that yellow fever was transmitted by a female *Aedes aegypti* mosquito. The mosquito feeds on an infected individual and spreads yellow fever once it bites the non-immune individual. It is at least a 12 day incubation period from the mosquito's initial exposure to the illness, to the time the female is infectious and develops the illness within her body, to the time the victim receives the bite from the infectious mosquito, to when symptoms will begin. Fomites, items such as bedding and clothing, do not spread yellow fever. They also found that a victim usually created enough immunity from their initial contraction of yellow fever, that it usually would not contract it a second time, if recovered from the first. Later, upon further investigation, they concluded that blood of an infected person could pass through a Pasteur filter and still be infectious. This was the first known filterable virus that caused a human infection.

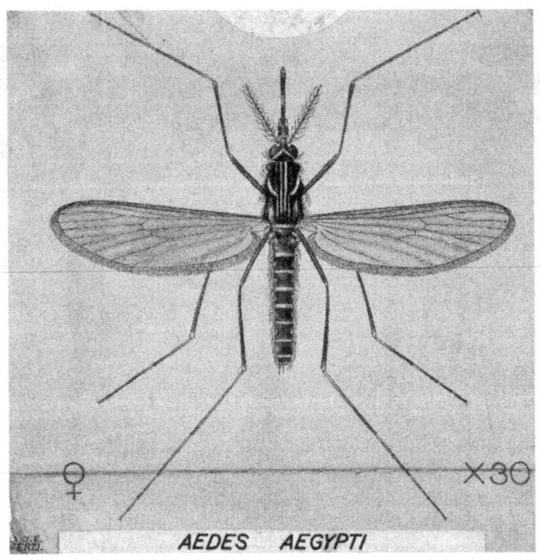

Figure – Aedes aegypti Mosquito

Reed wrote on these findings in his second paper, "The Etiology of Yellow Fever — An Additional Note," and presented them at the Pan-American Medical Congress in Havana in February of 1901. At the conference, Walter Reed was received warmly and wrote to his wife, "I received dozens of the warmest kinds of handshakes from Cuban, Spanish, Mexican, South American, and North American physicians, men whom I had not even met. The hall was crowded and the doors even packed with listeners. It was indeed a signal triumph for our work." Even with the excitement of the conclusion of all his hard work, Walter Reed goes on in the same letter, "[I] care more for what my sweet wifie & daughter care, think, and say, than for the applause of all of the rest of the world!" Walter Reed was ready to get back home to his family. This was his last letter he sent home before he boarded the boat back to Washington, DC. This marked the conclusion of the primary clinical work of the US Army Yellow Fever Commission.

CHAPTER 7

An Unexpected Death

History had been made with the scientific findings of the US Army Yellow Fever Commission, and millions of lives and dollars would be saved. The first implementations of these findings were used in Cuba. This information was put in the hands of General Leonard Wood, the Military Governor of Cuba, and Major William Crawford Gorgas, the Chief Sanitary Officer for the Department of Cuba. Major Gorgas organized efforts to rid Cuba of this pestilence. First, all patients possibly ill with yellow fever were to be kept behind a screen, as to not be accessible to mosquitoes. Second, chemicals were sprayed to kill adult mosquitoes in homes and buildings. Third, all standing water was drained, especially those around people, so that mosquitoes could not breed. Gorgas's work rid Cuba of its yellow fever problem, which had been plaguing the country for nearly fifty years, within three months! This was amazing, considering many modern day discoveries take decades to implement!

Now it was time to share with the rest of the world what the US Army Yellow Fever Commission had discovered. In February of 1901, Walter Reed began to share with the medical world all that they had learned about yellow fever. He resumed his teaching duties at the Army Medical School and at the Columbian University Medical School, and also continued to write and speak on yellow fever. Due to his work on yellow fever, he received honorary degrees from Harvard University and the University of Michigan in the summer of 1902. In addition, in November of 1902, he was named Librarian of the Surgeon General's Library. He was slated to become a Lieutenant Colonel within a few months. Walter was always working very hard, fulfilling his multiple professional duties.

In November of 1902, Walter Reed became ill and was unable to teach his evening class at the Columbian University. Two days later, at work, he was still feeling ill and his close friend, Major William C. Borden, sent him home. They spoke about Walter's symptoms and agreed that it was likely his appendix and he might need surgery. By Sunday night, Walter was doing much worse. Monday morning he was taken to the Army hospital. On November 17, he underwent surgery, performed by Major Borden, where he removed his ruptured appendix. His prognosis was a healthy recovery but that did not come to pass. Shortly after, on November 23, he died, at the age of 51, due to peritonitis that had developed.

His funeral took place at St. Thomas Church near Dupont Circle in Washington, DC on November 25, 1902. It was an affair in Washington and many high ranking military officers were in attendance, as well as many renowned physicians and scientists. Oddly enough, Walter Reed's wife was not in attendance, possibly due to illness and despair over losing her dear husband.

Walter Reed was laid to rest in Arlington National Cemetery. In the unofficial hospital section, Section 3, amid many other medical professionals, Walter Reed was buried. His head stone read, "He gave to man control of that dreadful scourge yellow fever." The United States military and the medical field felt a great loss from this man and his untimely, early death. At the peak of his scientific and medical career, it was over. Nonetheless, Walter Reed's legacy lives on in many areas.

The Walter Reed Memorial Association was formed shortly after his death, to provide for his widow and daughter as well as create a memorial for Dr. Walter Reed. Emilie Reed lived for forty-eight more years and died at the age of 94 on July 23, 1950. His daughter, Blossom Reed, married for a short time but never had any children. She lived in Pennsylvania with her mother. Blossom Reed died on August 22, 1964.

Lawrence Reed followed in his father's footsteps and served in the United States Army. Joining the enlisted ranks, he eventually became an officer and served for over 40 years. He retired as a major general. He also served as the Inspector General of the Army from 1935 to 1939. He died on May 1, 1956. Emilie, Blossom, and Lawrence are all buried in the Arlington National Cemetery.

CHAPTER 8

Final Yellow Fever Epidemic in the United States

When Walter Reed died, the developments regarding yellow fever were still rather new in the scientific and medical communities. Although there was proof regarding the US Army Yellow Fever Commission's findings, many were still skeptical of its truth, especially in the United States. Only three years after Walter Reed's death, an epidemic of yellow fever broke out in New Orleans.

Rather than adopting the new methods, as health officials were still skeptical, they treated the epidemic as they would have in the past. This was done through a strict quarantine system, the fumigation of ships, and the sanitation of clothing and bedding on board. These techniques did not prevent yellow fever, however, so it was no coincidence that the epidemic continued to spread and the numbers of deaths increased. In a single day, one hundred people fell victim to the illness. Even the Archbishop of the St. Louis Cathedral in New Orleans died of yellow fever. Finally, out of desperation, city officials decided to use new methods to treat the epidemic, such as the ones that had been implemented in Cuba and had been successful.

First, any areas of standing water or breeding grounds for mosquitoes were drained. If it was a cistern, kerosene was poured on the top of the surface to interfere with mosquito breeding, or a screen was placed over the opening. Second, yellow fever patients were kept inside with screens around them, thus keeping mosquitoes from feeding on them and then spreading their infected blood to healthy individuals. Finally, houses and buildings were sprayed for mosquitoes. As these implementations were strictly put into place, the epidemic began to slow.

Officials were still concerned, however, and had used up their local funds. Out of desperation and concern, national officials were contacted to help with the yellow fever epidemic. The US Public Health and Marine Hospital Service, now the United States Public Health Service, was brought in. They were able to further enforce and inspect the policies the local government had put into place. By early fall, the epidemic had ended, leaving in its wake a death toll of over 400 people and many more that had contracted the illness. This was the first time in US history that a yellow fever epidemic had ended due to intervention rather than just the first frost. Many credit this as the first and most successful public health campaign in the United States. This was wonderful news for our nation which had been plagued with yellow fever epidemics since its founding.

CHAPTER 9

Legacy

The most illustrious legacy left by Dr. Walter Reed is the Walter Reed Army Medical Center. Seven years after Walter Reed's death, the Walter Reed General Hospital in Washington, DC opened. This facility would become one of Walter Reed's most notable legacies and namesakes, serving thousands of wounded soldiers as well as many dignitaries and presidents. The project was spearheaded by Major William C. Borden, who was Reed's friend and personal doctor as well as the surgeon that had operated on him before he died. Reed had been the only appendectomy patient that Borden had ever lost and he was distraught. This distress birthed a desire to truly honor Walter Reed. "Borden's Dream," as it became called, was to have the Army Medical Museum, the Army Medical School, and a hospital all located on one campus. He faced barriers and complications but pushed through them and let no one detour him from his goal. He even worked, personally, on the funding of this massive project.

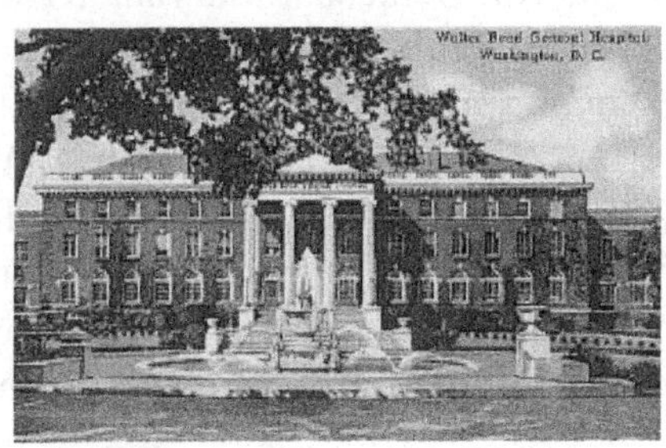

Figure – Walter Reed General Hospital circa 1930s

May 1, 1909, the Walter Reed General Hospital saw its first patients. In 1923, the Army Medical School moved to the same site. In 1951, on the 100th year anniversary of Walter Reed's birth, the name of the installation was changed to the Walter Reed Army Medical Center. The Walter Reed Army Institute of Research, the successor to the Army Medical School, was renamed in 1953. Today it is the largest biomedical research facility managed by the Department of Defense. In 1966, following Blossom Reed's death, the Walter Reed Memorial Association, as one of its final acts, had a bronze bust of Walter Reed created. President Eisenhower revealed a memorial and this bronze bust of Walter Reed on the grounds of Walter Reed Army Medical Center in a large ceremony. In 1971, the National Museum of Health and Medicine moved to the campus as well. After several years of planning, in 1972, construction began on the new Walter Reed Army Medical Center hospital facility. This facility was dedicated in 1977. Over the years, additional facilities were built and the hospital capacity grew to about 250 beds, serving approximately 150,000 soldiers, their family members, and military retirees. In 2005, the Base Realignment and Closure Act mandated the merger of Walter Reed Army Medical Center with the National Naval Medical Center in Bethesda, Maryland. The Army unit colors were cased on July 27, 2011. The National Colors were lowered over Walter Reed Army Medical Center for the final time at noon on September 15, 2011. As this facility closed, Walter Reed National Military Medical Center, Bethesda officially opened with the dedication ceremony occurring on November 10, 2011. This facility continues to operate today as a joint military operation that has an Army

General as the Director and a Navy Captain as the Chief of Staff. In addition, Army, Navy, and Air Force leadership is integrated throughout the entire Chain of Command.

Additionally, in 1996, the Walter Reed Society was established to preserve Reed's legacy. The society's mission statement states: "The Society's vision is to serve as a strong voluntary organization — comprising individuals affiliated with the original Walter Reed Army Medical Center and its successor organization, Walter Reed National Military Medical Center — which actively supports the institution, its people, and its legacy. The purpose of The Walter Reed Society, Inc. is to first, support activities and fund projects to benefit service members and staff at the medical center, particularly if associated with education, treatment, or research. Second, to provide good stewardship of the funds donated and grants awarded to assist service members and/or their family members, which are intended to provide them with help with unexpected financial needs and to provide them with specially identified equipment and services related to patient care at the medical center when other resources are not available. Finally, to seek to preserve the legacy of Walter Reed, the man and the institution named in his honor, by involving and communicating with the membership and friends of Walter Reed National Military Medical Center through educational activities, the newsletter, and the website. Membership in the Society is open to all military and civilian personnel who have associations with the medical center, to include patients, staff, those who attended any course of instruction at these institutions, providers of goods and services, friends and neighbors."

Walter Reed was also honored by Congress's enacting of the Army Register's Roll of Honor. This act entitled the listed individuals (or their survivors) to receive a Congressional Gold Medal and a monthly pension. This was the government's way of honoring and providing for those who sacrificed for the greater good. In 1929, Congress passed Public Law No. 858 to acknowledge Dr. Walter Reed's work regarding yellow fever. It read:

"Be it enacted by the Senate and House or Representatives of the United States of America in Congress assembled, That in special recognition of the high public service rendered and disabilities contracted in the interest of humanity and science as voluntary subjects for the experimentations during the yellow-fever investigations in Cuba, the Secretary of War, be, and he is hereby, authorized and directed to publish annually in the Army Register a roll of honor on which shall be carried the following names: Walter Reed, James Carroll, Jesse W. Lazear, Aristides Agramonte, James H. Andrus, John R. Bullard, A.W. Covington, William H. Dean, Wallace W. Forbes, Levi E. Folk, Paul Hamann, James L. Hanberry, Warren G. Jernegan, John R. Kissinger, John J. Moran, William Olsen, Charles G. Sonntag, Clyde L. West, Doctor R.P. Cook, Thomas M. England, James Hildebrand, and Edward Weatherwalks." In 1957, this act was amended and Gustaf E. Lambert and Roger P. Ames were added.

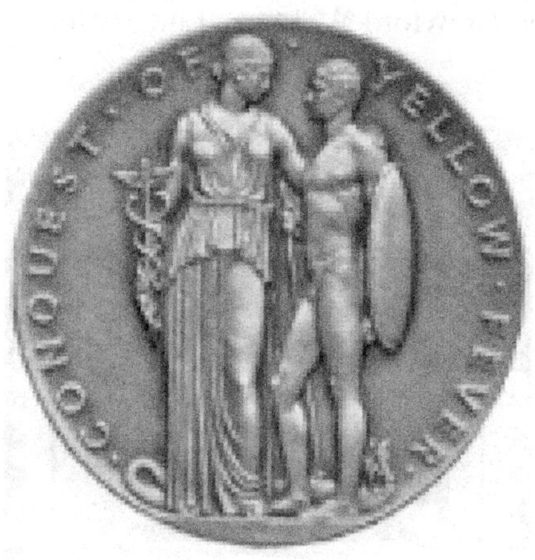

Figure – Congressional Gold Medal

Moreover, Walter Reed's life has been honored by the restoration and preservation of his birth home. In 1973, Walter Reed's birthplace was added to the National Register of Historic Places. The Virginia Medical Society restored the two bedroom cottage in Gloucester County, Virginia in 1927. It was remodeled again in 1970. In May 2013, stewardship of the Walter Reed Birthplace was transferred to the Gloucester Preservation Foundation. It is open to the public and can still be visited today. For further visitor information, contact the Gloucester Preservation Foundation.

In 1940, Walter Reed was pictured on a United States five cent postage stamp. The US Post Office issued a set of 35 stamps, issued over the course of approximately ten months, commemorating America's famous Authors, Poets, Educators, Scientists, Composers, Artists and Inventors. The other Scientists featured along with Walter Reed were John James

Audubon, Dr. Crawford W. Long, Luther Burbank, and Jane Addams.

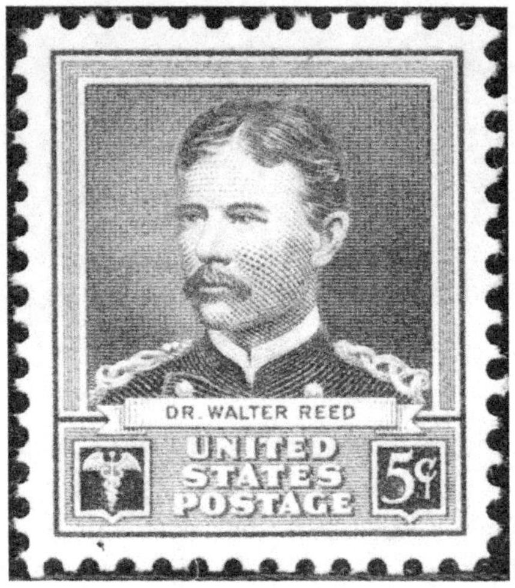

Figure – Five-cent Dr. Walter Reed Stamp

In 1945, Reed was elected to the Hall of Fame of Great Americans at New York University. He was the first physician bestowed this honor. The Hall of Fame for Great Americans is an outdoor sculpture gallery, located on the grounds of Bronx Community College in the Bronx, New York City. To be eligible for nomination, a person must have been a native born or naturalized citizen of the United States, must have been dead for 25 years, and must have made a major contribution to the economic, political, or cultural life of the nation. Nominees were elected by a simple majority vote. William C. Gorgas was also elected to the Hall of Fame in 1950.

Furthermore, The Walter Reed Medal is awarded every third year to recognize distinguished accomplishments in the field of tropical medicine by the American Society of Tropical Medicine and Hygiene. The first award was made in 1936 to Mrs. Walter Reed and to the Rockefeller Foundation. Thirty-three individuals have since received the same award, including Dr. Carlos Finlay, posthumously.

Finally, multiple television documentaries, movies, and screenplays have been written featuring Walter Reed and his scientific discoveries. The most notable was the movie *Yellow Jack,* from 1938, where the actor Lewis Stone played the role of Walter Reed.

Credits and Acknowledgments

All photos are from the public domain. I would like to thank Doug West (editor), Lisa Zahn, Luan Sparks, and Harjit S. Sandhu for their help in preparation of the book. Finally, thank you to my husband, Walter DeLong, for his support and encouragement throughout this process.

Further Reading

Bean, William B. *Walter Reed*. University Press of Virginia. 1982.

Wood, L. N. *Walter Reed – Doctor in Uniform*. Julian Messner, Inc. 1943.

Writer, Jim and John R. Pierce. *Yellow Jack – How Yellow Fever Ravaged America and Walter Reed Discovered Its Deadly Secrets*. John Wiley & Sons, Inc. 2005.

About the Author

Erin DeLong is a wife, mother, writer, and runner. Erin has a Bachelor's degree in Human and Community Services with minors in community health and health administration from New Mexico State University. She also served in the United States Army and spent time overseas serving with the 31st Combat Support Hospital. She loves volunteering in her church and community, being outside, and spending time at home with her four boys and husband.

Follow the book series on Facebook at: https://www.facebook.com/30minutebooks.

Additional Books in the "30 Minute Book Series"

A Short Biography of the Scientist Sir Isaac Newton

A Short Biography of the Astronomer Edwin Hubble

Galileo Galilei – A Short Biography

Benjamin Franklin – A Short Biography

The American Revolutionary War – A Short History

The Astronomer Cecilia Payne-Gaposchkin – A Short Biography

Index

Made in the USA
Monee, IL
07 July 2026

56551360R00036